Houda Boukhrissa

# Viral hepatitis E, clinical, diagnostic and therapeutic aspects

Houda Boukhrissa

# Viral hepatitis E, clinical, diagnostic and therapeutic aspects

ScienciaScripts

This book is a translation from the original published under ISBN 978-620-6-71222-0.

Publisher:
Sciencia Scripts
is a trademark of
Dodo Books Indian Ocean Ltd. and OmniScriptum S.R.L publishing group

120 High Road, East Finchley, London, N2 9ED, United Kingdom
Str. Armeneasca 28/1, office 1, Chisinau MD-2012, Republic of Moldova, Europe
Printed at: see last page
**ISBN: 978-620-7-71454-4**

# Viral hepatitis E

# Clinical, diagnostic and therapeutic aspects

# Table of Contents

# I. INTRODUCTION

Hepatitis E virus (HEV) is one of the main causes of acute viral hepatitis worldwide [1]. Belonging to the Hepeviridae family, this single-stranded RNA virus is transmitted mainly via the faecal-oral route, making it a major health concern in regions where sanitation is poor and access to drinking water limited [2]. The infection is endemic in many developing countries in Asia, Africa and Central America, with an estimated 20 million cases each year [3]. Although less frequent, sporadic cases linked to travel to endemic areas or ingestion of contaminated food are regularly reported in industrialised nations [4]. There are currently eight genotypes of HEV, of which 1 and 2 are strictly human pathogens, while 3 and 4 are zoonotic in nature, finding their reservoirs in various animal species such as domestic and wild swine and deer [5]. While human-to-human transmission via the faecal-oral and blood-borne routes, as well as maternal-foetal transmission, has been confirmed, the methods of zoonotic contamination remain to be specified [6]. In most cases, HEV causes an acute form of the disease that resolves spontaneously, with rapid viral clearance. However, the disease can progress to a fulminant form, with a mortality rate of between 1% and 4% in the general population. This severe form is more common in pregnant women and people with chronic liver disease. A particularly high mortality rate of 15-20% has been classically described in pregnant women during epidemic outbreaks [7]. Recent data suggest that acute infection may progress to a chronic form in various immunocompromised situations (organ transplantation, haematological malignancy and human immunodeficiency virus infection), which may be complicated by cirrhosis, sometimes rapidly progressive [8]. Extra-hepatic manifestations, especially neurological, have recently been reported [9].

Hepatitis E is generally under-diagnosed due to a lack of awareness among doctors in many countries. Major advances in serological and molecular tests mean that the diagnosis can be made reliably in both immunocompetent and immunosuppressed patients [10]. Diagnosis should be considered in the event of any unexplained acute hepatic cytolysis, and is based on the detection of anti-HEV immunoglobulin M (IgM). Because serological tests are less sensitive in immunocompromised patients, testing for HEV RNA in blood or stools is essential[11].

Treatment of chronic hepatitis E with ribavirin monotherapy has proved effective in immunocompromised patients and is currently widely recommended. Its real benefit in acute forms has not yet been established [12]. An effective, well-tolerated vaccine was developed in 2011 and is licensed in China. It could be of interest for at-risk populations, particularly patients with established cirrhosis and travellers to endemic areas [13,14].

## II. EPIDEMIOLOGY

The hepatitis E virus (HEV) was discovered in 1983 during an unexplained outbreak of hepatitis in a Soviet military camp in Afghanistan [15]. A member of the research team ingested a contaminated faecal extract from infected soldiers, which enabled electron microscopy to recognise the new virus in his faeces [16].

Transmission of HEV is mainly faecal-oral, via ingestion of water or food contaminated with infected faeces [15]. However, other routes are possible, such as blood transmission, notably by transfusion or during medical procedures [10]. Maternal-foetal transmission and human-to-human transmission through close contact have also been reported [17].

In developing countries, the spread of hepatitis E is mainly due to the consumption of contaminated water during flash floods, while in developed countries, sporadic cases are mainly linked to the consumption of contaminated food products of animal origin [18]. HEV genotypes 1 and 2, which are responsible for epidemics in poor countries, are endemic in Asia, Africa, Latin America and the Middle East, with high attack rates in young adults [19]. The regions most affected are in South and South-East Asia, sub-Saharan Africa and some parts of Central America. Zoonotic genotypes 3 and 4 predominate in developed countries, where pig infection is the main reservoir. Although sporadic, these cases are more frequent in the elderly, haemodialysis patients and immunocompromised individuals [18]. Finally, zoonotic spread of genotype 7 (Orthohepevirus C) by rodents has recently been observed, suggesting a potential reservoir that is as yet unknown [18].

## III. PATHOPHYSIOLOGY

The mechanisms involved in the pathogenicity of HEV are poorly characterised. It seems that the damage caused by the virus is due more to a cytotoxic immune response than to a direct cytopathogenic effect of the virus. Indeed, viremia precedes biochemical and histopathological manifestations by several days, and there is no evidence of a direct cytopathogenic effect of the virus [20].

Several factors have been implicated in the pathogenesis, either host-related, such as pregnancy, chronic liver disease and immunosuppression, or virus-related. According to epidemiological, clinical and experimental observations, HEV 1 and 2 are more virulent than HEV 3 and 4, although HEV 4 appears to be associated with more severe manifestations than HEV 3 [21,22].

There are still very few studies looking at the anti-HEV immune response.

### 1. Immune response in the acute stage of hepatitis

#### 1.1 Innate immune response

During acute hepatitis E, it has been shown that the number of natural killer (NK) and natural killer T (NKT) cells present in the peripheral blood was reduced compared with the number observed in healthy controls [23]. The low peripheral immune response observed is thought to be linked to the migration and sequestration of immune cells in the liver. Interleukin (IL)-1 and IL-2 show higher serum concentrations during the inflammatory phase in patients with acute hepatitis E, suggesting their involvement in pathogenesis [20].

**1.2 Adaptive immune response**

**1.2.1 Humoral response**

The anti-HEV humoral response is detectable from the onset of symptoms. IgM appears early in the course of the disease. IgG is detected shortly after IgM. Their titre increases during the acute phase and convalescence. The antibodies secreted are directed against the proteins encoded by ORF1, the capsid protein encoded by ORF2 and the protein encoded by ORF3[20].

**1.2.2 Cellular response**

Hepatic recruitment of CD8+ T lymphocytes during acute hepatitis E has been observed in studies of liver biopsies from infected patients. The cell-mediated immune response therefore appears to be essential for eradicating the virus. In immunocompromised patients, impairment of this T response leads to the persistence of HEV [24].

**2. Immune response and severity of HEV infection**

**2.1 Fulminant hepatitis**

In fulminant hepatitis E, serum levels of anti-HEV IgM and IgG are higher than those observed in uncomplicated hepatitis E. A higher frequency of CD4 T cells and CD8 T cells was found in the liver. Low levels of IFN (interferon) and TNF (tumour necrosis factor) secretion were also found in these patients. Thus, a Th2 type response (T helpers) associated with low IFN levels seems to favour the development of fulminant hepatitis and the death of the patient [128]. NF-KB is a dimeric transcription factor with several cellular roles, including liver regeneration. A mouse lacking the p65 component of NF-BK showed generalised apoptosis of the liver. The same deficiency was observed in pregnant women suffering from fulminant forms of hepatitis B, C and E viruses. The absence of NF-BK p65 is therefore responsible for fulminant liver damage [25].

## 2.2 The special case of pregnant women

Several pathophysiological hypotheses have been put forward to explain the severity of infection at the end of pregnancy. An immunological hypothesis has been put forward, with an imbalance in the Th1/Th2 cell-mediated immune balance; an increase in the Th2 response and a decrease in Th1, not found in non-pregnant women. In addition, variations in hormone levels (increased progesterone, oestrogen and chronic human gonadotropin) promote lymphocyte apoptosis and viral replication [25]. In addition to immunological factors, virological factors may also be involved. Higher viral loads are found in pregnant women with fulminant hepatitis compared with pregnant women with an uncomplicated form. The viruses isolated all belong to HEV1, and the influence of other genotypes has not been studied [26]. Other factors, such as nutritional status and folic acid deficiency, can affect the immune response and increase the risk of HEV infection in pregnant women [27]. Thus, a combination of immunological, hormonal and virological factors could explain the severity of fulminant hepatitis in pregnant women in endemic regions. However, the above hypotheses do not fully explain the absence of fulminant hepatitis in pregnant women in industrialised countries. Further studies are underway to understand the variability in the severity of acute hepatitis E in different regions [25].

## 3. Mechanisms of HEV persistence in immunocompromised patients

### 3.1 Host factors

Available data suggest that the level of immunosuppression plays a very important role, but the nature of the innate or adaptive immune responses whose alteration leads to chronicity has not yet been identified. Specific anti-HEV CD4/T CD8 T responses and neutralising antibodies are the subject of several studies, as is the existence of genetic determinants associated with HEV persistence [28].

## 3.2 Viral factors

The chronic course has been almost exclusively caused by HEV 3 and 4. Until recently, persistent infections due to HEV 7 have been described. Subtype differences may exist within HEV 3. Most chronic hepatitis E cases described to date involve subtypes 3f and 3c. However, this may simply reflect the preponderance of these subtypes in continental Europe [29].

## IV. ANATOMOPATHOLOGY

There are few histological studies in the literature. Most of those published are the result of analyses carried out during major hepatitis E epidemics in developing countries, and are very often post-mortem analyses [30]. Two forms of acute hepatitis, known as classical and cholestatic, may be observed.

The classic form is the most common, with generally marked necrotic-inflammatory activity. Hepatocyte necrosis is confluent or focal, in the form of isolated acetowhite bodies or ballooning hepatocytes, associated with polymorphous and lymphocytic inflammation of the portal and mixed parenchymal tissues.

The cholestatic form combines cholangiolar proliferation with a polymorphous inflammatory infiltrate of the portal spaces and lobules.
These two forms have also been described in patients with hepatitis E from non-endemic countries [31].

# V.  CLINIC

## 1. Acute forms

The clinical presentation of acute hepatitis E is similar to that of acute hepatitis caused by other hepatotropic viruses. In endemic areas, hepatitis E mainly affects adolescents and young adults. In non-endemic areas, it mainly affects adults over the age of 50, where it is often misdiagnosed as autoimmune or drug-induced hepatitis [32]. The clinical spectrum is broad, ranging from mild or asymptomatic to fulminant forms.

### 1.1 Common icteric form

Present in 10-50% of cases, it presents as acute cytolytic hepatitis with a favourable outcome [10].

### 1.1.1.  Incubation period :

The incubation period varies from 15 to 60 days, with an average of 40 days. This approximation is based on the results of infection in two volunteers and numerous experiments on *cynomolgus* monkeys [21].

### 1.1.2.  Prodromal phase :

The most common symptoms are flu-like, with fever or feverishness (58%), chills, headache, asthenia, anorexia, myalgia and joint pain. In half the cases, the patient complains of digestive problems, often moderate, such as epigastric pain or pain in the right hypochondrium, vomiting and diarrhoea. In a small number of patients, a skin rash of various types develops, in the form of maculopapular erythema or urticaria. This pre-icteric phase lasts an average of 3 to 7 days; it is sometimes absent, sometimes brief, and can sometimes persist for up to two weeks [32].

### 1.1.3 State phase :

The beginning of the icteric phase is marked by the gradual appearance of jaundice, which reaches its peak in four to eight days and varies in intensity from one patient to another. Urine is scanty and dark. Stools are normal or discoloured. The functional and general signs of the pre-ictal period persist for one or two weeks, then gradually diminish. Asthenia is accompanied by various digestive clinical signs such as nausea, vomiting, abdominal pain and anorexia. Some patients also present with hyperthermia, which is generally moderate. Finally, some studies report more atypical symptoms such as diarrhoea, pruritus and arthralgia. Neurological symptoms such as encephalitis or Guillain-Barré syndrome are sometimes found [33]. At this stage, the physical examination may be normal or may reveal small lymphadenopathies (particularly in the posterior cervical region). In about half of patients, the liver is slightly enlarged and often tender to palpation. Jaundice gradually diminishes. The average duration is 2 to 6 weeks [32].

### 1.1.4 Evolution :

The course of this disease is usually benign, and it generally recovers spontaneously and without sequelae after 2 to 4 weeks. Jaundice gradually diminishes, asthenia generally disappears little by little with the jaundice, stools regain their colour and appetite gradually returns. However, malaise, tiredness and fatigue may persist for longer. In all cases, clinical and biochemical recovery usually occurs in less than six months [34].

## 1.2 Anicteric and asymptomatic forms

Nearly half of all cases are asymptomatic or pauci-symptomatic. Clinical symptoms, in particular asthenia and arthralgias, are identical to those of the icteric form, with the exception of jaundice. The biochemical abnormalities, in particular the increase in transaminases, are identical, with the obvious exception of hyperbilirubinaemia [35].

## 1.3 Reactivation, reinfection and relapse

Reactivation of HEV has been suggested on the basis of two clinical cases. In the first case, viremia reappeared 14 weeks after allografting in a patient with acute lymphocytic leukaemia. In the second case, viremia reappeared seven weeks after allogeneic transplantation in a patient with acute myeloid leukaemia. However, these two studies do not mention whether the virus was still detectable in the faeces at the time of apparent recovery. No reactivation was observed in patients who had received stem cell transplants or in patients with solid organ transplants [36].

Reinfections appear to be frequent and may lead to the development of a new infection. Relapses are exceptional [22].

## 1.4 Cholestatic forms

The cholestatic form may occur secondary to a common form, with intense cholestasis, dark jaundice and intense pruritus. Biologically, cholestasis predominates, with significant elevation of alkaline phosphatases, and cytolysis may even have disappeared, raising possible diagnostic problems with extra-hepatic cholestasis. Progression is generally slow, taking 3 to 4 months, but recovery is usually complete [37].

## 1.5 Fulminant forms

This is the most serious form. In 1 to 2% of cases, the acute form is complicated by a fulminant form with acute hepatocellular failure (AHF), leading to massive destruction of the liver parenchyma with hepatocyte necrosis and liver atrophy [30]. In this case, the patient's vital prognosis is at stake because there is no specific treatment, and liver transplantation is often the only solution. The incidence rate of fulminant forms is considerably higher in pregnant women during the third trimester, reaching 20%. The mortality rate is over 20% [38]. In industrialised countries, fulminant hepatitis has not been observed in pregnant women, but it occurs with a high frequency (around 10%) in people with underlying liver disease. Cases of fulminant hepatitis E in pregnant women in non-endemic areas have occurred following a stay in an endemic area [39]. Clinically, the picture is characterised by increasingly intense jaundice, deterioration in liver function (in particular the synthesis of coagulation factors), encephalopathy and finally coma and multi-visceral failure [32].

## 1.6 Special situations

### 1.6.1 Hepatitis E and chronic liver disease

HEV is an aggravating factor in chronic liver disease. Several articles have described an exacerbation of pre-existing liver disease in the event of superinfection by HEV, whether the primary disease was due to alcohol or to another virus with hepatic tropism (HBV, HCV)[40]. This worsening is most often characterised by a very marked rise in liver cytolysis parameters and sometimes even by severe decompensation manifested by ascites and more or less pronounced hepatic encephalopathy[32]. In the absence of liver transplantation, the course is unfavourable, with a mortality rate of 70% in patients infected with HEV1[41]. Liver histology is inconclusive in patients with underlying cirrhosis, and ribavirin-based treatment can, in some cases, avoid the need for a liver transplant [22].

### 1.6.2 Hepatitis E and pregnancy

Most of the data on clinical manifestations in pregnant women have been recorded in Asia, mainly India, and Africa, where the majority of viral hepatitis cases described in pregnant women are linked to HEV (60% of cases)[42]. Previous epidemiological studies carried out in the absence of specific serological and virological tools showed a higher frequency and severity of NANB enteric hepatitis in pregnant women. Since then, new serological studies have confirmed an incidence rate of 20% and a case-fatality rate of between 20 and 40% when infection occurs during the third trimester of pregnancy [38]. Initially, the clinical features do not differ from those of non-pregnant women. However, after a short period, these clinical manifestations may progress to HAI with disseminated intravascular coagulation, encephalopathy and cerebral oedema. The rate of occurrence of these complications can be as high as 70% in women infected with HEV1. In addition, observational studies have shown that, among pregnant women, HEV has a higher rate of fatal HAI than other known viral hepatitis agents[32]. Fetal and/or maternal mortality depends on the viral load and the severity of symptoms. It has been estimated that HEV infection may be responsible for between 2,400 and 3,000 deaths at birth each year, in addition to foetal deaths linked to maternal mortality. Premature delivery, low birth weight and death of the newborn are observed in 25% to 56% of cases[42]. Surprisingly, this situation is different in Egypt, where HEV infection in pregnant women is not associated with high mortality. Some authors suggest a lower virulence of genotype 1 under predominant type 3 [43]. Hepatitis E in pregnant women is very rare in developed countries, where the course of the disease is almost unknown due to the small number of cases. In recent years, sporadic indigenous cases caused by HEV3 and HEV4 have been reported. A study was carried out in France to assess the prevalence of infection during pregnancy. Of the 315 pregnant women taking part, the prevalence of HEV was 7.74%. No deaths were observed, suggesting a lower virulence of the genotype involved[25].

## 2. Chronic forms

HEV infection used to be considered strictly acute in nature, but a progression to chronicity, defined by the persistence of viremia for more than six months, has recently been demonstrated in various situations of immunosuppression: solid organ transplantation, including in children [44], haematological diseases [45] and HIV infection [46]. The first case described was that of a patient with lymphoma treated with chemotherapy and a bone marrow allograft [45], in whom faecal excretion of the virus persisted for 10 months. Since then, several other cases have been reported in France and Japan [8]. The acute infection preceding the chronic phase is often mild or asymptomatic, dominated by isolated asthenia. It is often discovered when moderate and fluctuating hypertransaminasemia occurs[11]. The diagnosis is made when HEV RNA is detected for more than 6 months, with or without the presence of anti-HEV IgG and IgM (a frequent defect in seroconversion). Testing for HEV RNA in blood and faeces should therefore be carried out systematically if chronic hepatitis E is suspected, including when transaminase levels are subnormal and fluctuating, even in the absence of anti-HEV IgG and IgM[11]. The disease may progress to fibrosis. The onset of cirrhosis is sometimes rapid and may necessitate a new liver transplant in previously transplanted patients [44]. To date, only two cases of chronic hepatitis E in immunocompetent individuals have been reported[47,48].

## 2.1 Transplant patients

Transplant patients, particularly kidney and liver transplant patients, are the main group at risk. Acute hepatitis E becomes chronic in almost two-thirds of these patients. The risk factors for chronicity are a short time between transplantation and HEV infection, low platelet and lymphocyte levels, particularly CD2, CD3 and CD4, and the prescription of tracrolimus as an immunosuppressant (vs ciclosporin) [28]. Rapidly progressive cirrhosis has been described within 12 to 36 months. The fibrosis score between two biopsies taken a mean of two years apart increased significantly by one Metavir unit (from 1 to 2). This compares with $0.09 \pm 0.03$ Metavir units/year in HCV-infected kidney transplant recipients. These data suggest that HEV infection in renal transplant recipients may be more severe than HCV infection [44].

## 2.2 Haematological diseases

The development of chronic HEV infection has been described in several lymphoma patients. The combined effects of haemopathy and treatment (high-dose corticosteroids, rituximab) are probably responsible for this development. When liver biopsies were performed, the histological lesions were either moderate or severe with a Metavir score of A3F3 [45]. Chronic HEV infection has recently been described in a patient with Hairy Cell Leukaemia who did not require treatment due to the very slow progression of the haemopathy.

### 2.2.3 HIV-infected patients

The first two cases of chronic hepatitis E observed in HIV-infected patients were described in 2009. Since then, new cases have been reported. The infection is often asymptomatic and is discovered when there is a disturbance in the liver function tests or when there is CD4 lymphopenia. Progression may be complicated by rapid onset of cirrhosis. An aetiological work-up should include an anti-HEV IgG and IgM assay and a search for the virus in blood and faeces, because of a seroconversion defect or delay frequently found in these patients. Natural elimination of HEV can be achieved after several months of effective antiretroviral treatment, concomitant with immune restoration [46].

### 3. Extra-hepatic manifestations

Extra-hepatic manifestations have been described during acute or chronic HEV infections.

### 3.1 Neurological symptoms

Most frequently described (5.5% of patients with acute and chronic infection), reported manifestations include Guillain-Barré syndrome, meningoencephalitis or neuritis. A bilateral pyramidal syndrome associated with peripheral neuropathy has been described in a renal transplant patient with chronic hepatitis E. Analysis of viral quasispecies in serum and cerebrospinal fluid was consistent with the emergence of neurotropic variants [33]. A large case-control study confirmed that 5% of patients with Guillain-Barré syndrome had acute hepatitis E [49].

### 3.2 Pancreatic involvement

Several cases of pancreatitis have been reported. Symptoms usually develop in the second or third week after the onset of jaundice and disappear spontaneously. Acute pancreatitis has only been reported in countries endemic for HEV 1[50].

### 3.3 Haematological manifestations

Thrombocytopenia and haemolytic anaemia have been described in countries both endemic and non-endemic for HEV. A case of Henoch-Schonlein purpura in a child has also been reported [51].

### 3.4 Kidney disorders

In solid organ transplant patients, a decrease in glomerular filtration rate has been observed in cases of HEV3 infection. Some cases of membrane glomerulonephritis and cryoglobulinemia have also been reported [44].

### 3.5 Rheumatological symptoms
Cases of acute polyarthritis revealing hepatitis E have been reported [52].

# VI. DIAGNOSTIC

## 1. Non-specific biological diagnosis

### 1.1 Liver function tests

Acute hepatitis should be suspected if there is a significant rise in serum transaminase activity, mainly alanine aminotransferase (ALT), whether or not associated with jaundice [53]. The increase in ALT generally precedes the onset of symptoms by around 10 days and reaches a peak towards the end of the first clinical week. The observed peak can reach very high values, up to 4100 IU/L, but is more often around 700-800 IU/L. This peak is monophasic and coincides with the onset of jaundice, as is the case for most viral hepatitis. Once the peak has been reached, serum transaminase and bilirubin levels begin to fall, returning to normal within 2 months in the majority of patients [54]. Alkaline phosphatase levels are normal or moderately elevated (less than 2 times the upper limit of normal), except in cholestatic forms where hyperphosphatasemia may be observed. Gamma glutamyl transpeptidase (yGT) activity is moderately elevated. Prothrombin time and prothrombin complex elements are moderately disturbed in common forms [54].

### 1.2 Blood tests

Leukopenia with neutropenia is sometimes observed. Quite frequently, serum iron is elevated; this hypersideraemia is attributed to necrosis of the hepatocytes, which release the iron they contain into the plasma [53].

## 2. Virological diagnosis

### 2.1 Indirect diagnosis

Indirect virological diagnosis reveals the humoral immune response, and the anti-HEV antibodies sought are routinely IgG and IgM. They are produced at different times during infection and can help to date contamination (Figure 7).

The presence of anti-HEV IgM is the key marker of acute infection. It appears on average 2 to 3 weeks before the first clinical signs. Their serum concentration peaks at the time of the ALT peak, i.e. during jaundice. IgM then gradually disappears over a period of 2 weeks to 3 months (sometimes 4 to 6 months)[10].

IgG appears shortly after IgM, and is detected in serum several days after the appearance of IgM. Their titre increases at the end of the clinical phase, then tends to fall slightly during convalescence, and they usually persist for several years. In Kashmir, researchers carried out serological follow-up of 320 people with hepatitis E. 50% of cases had detectable anti-HEV IgG 14 years after infection. In another short-term follow-up study, the researchers found that 100% of people retained anti-HEV IgG 3 years later [36]. Overall, IgG declines slowly in most patients over time, but the minimum titre required for protection is unknown [55].

The techniques used are: immunofluorescence, immunochromatography and immunoenzymology (ELISA and western blot). The existence of a single serotype means that proteins isolated from HEV 1 and 2 can be used to test for HEV antibodies, regardless of the genotype that caused the infection [11].

• IgM detection techniques: enzyme immunoassay techniques are the most widely used. Recent studies have shown that the commercial kits currently available have very good sensitivity (> 97% in immunocompetent patients > 85% in immunocompromised patients) and very good specificity (> %)[56].

In immunocompetent subjects, the lack of sensitivity of anti-HEV IgM is most often secondary to early infection (positive viremia with negative antibodies). The absence of seroconversion is possible and has been estimated at 1 to 4% of cases per year in China [57]. In immunocompromised patients, the serological diagnosis may be faulty, with delayed or even absent anti-HEV seroconversion. Acquired immunodepression inhibits the activation of T cells (NK cells, regulatory T lymphocytes) and compromises the anti-HEV response [58]. False positives are generally linked to cross-reactions in the presence of hyperimmune sera (non-specific polyclonal reaction linked to an acute infection of another origin): CMV or EBV infection [59].

• IgG detection technique: several enzyme-linked immunosorbent assays (ELISAs) can be used to detect IgG antibodies, with varying degrees of sensitivity. Studies show that the Wantai kit is more sensitive due to its lower detection limit for IgG antibodies (0.25 WHO units/L compared with 2.5 WHO units/L for the others)[60].

The detection of anti-HEV IgG alone does not confirm the recent nature of the viral infection, but it does indicate contact with the virus. In theory, a combined IgM-IgG positive test after an initial work-up showing only isolated anti-HEV IgM positivity is very strongly in favour of acute hepatitis E [11].

• The anti-HEV IgG avidity test measures the binding strength of IgG antigen-antibodies (Ag-Ac), enabling a recent infection (low Ag-Ac binding strength) to be distinguished from an old infection.

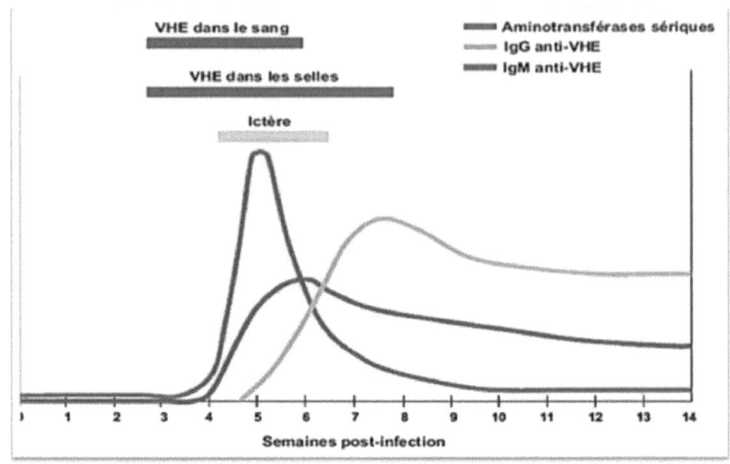


Figure 7: Changes in biological parameters during HEV infection [36].

## 2.2 Direct diagnosis

Experimental infection has shown that viral RNA is detected in the serum around the 22nd day post-inoculation, persists during the pre-ictal phase and then decreases during the icteric phase, disappearing at the time of the ALT peak [54]. In a natural infection, the relatively brief viremia (four weeks) occurs mainly during the prodromal phase and disappears when symptoms appear, but this pattern is not systematic. Some studies have reported prolonged viremia of 4 to 16 weeks [61].

Direct diagnosis is based on:

- Conventional or real-time RT-PCR, which consists of amplifying part of the HEV genome. Samples are either serum or supernatant from stool washing or liver tissue and bile [62]. Given the genotypic heterogeneity of HEV, this amplification is carried out on the most conserved genomic regions of ORF 1, 2 or 3 in order to guarantee the best diagnostic sensitivity [36].

• sequencing and therefore genotyping of strains for a molecular epidemiology approach.

• in vitro culture of the virus on cell lines is restricted to specialist laboratories due to its limited feasibility. Testing for viral antigens using a technique that detects HEV 1 and 4 capsid proteins [39].

The main limitations of virus detection are a narrow detection window and intermittent excretion [63]. Conversely, molecular biology can be used to diagnose rare cases of serologically silent hepatitis E in immunocompetent or immunocompromised patients [39]. In immunocompromised patients, HEV RNA testing is required in three situations: cytolysis without detection of anti-HEV IgM, to determine the risk of progression to chronic infection, and to monitor the efficacy of any treatment [64].

In practice, in endemic areas, the diagnosis must be made in the presence of any acute cytolytic non-A, non-B, non-C hepatitis. These areas correspond to developing countries, where serological tests are much less expensive than molecular biology techniques and therefore more affordable[65]. In industrialised countries, the diagnosis was traditionally based on the clinical presentation, the epidemic context or a recent history of a stay in an endemic area. It should now be considered in the presence of any acute hepatitis of unexplained origin, even if there is no evidence of endemic travel. In immunocompetent patients, the diagnosis of acute hepatitis E is usually made by detecting anti-HEV IgM. Since serological tests are less sensitive in immunocompromised patients, it is essential to test for viral RNA in plasma or stools [65].

# VII. TREATMENT

## 1. Curative treatment

### 1.1 Non-specific measures

#### 1.1.1 Common acute forms

The course of acute hepatitis E in immunocompetent patients is self-limiting in the majority of cases, and treatment is symptomatic only, with hospitalisation only indicated for patients unable to eat orally. Strict rest and a special diet are not necessary. Any additional hepatotoxic factors should be avoided, in particular paracetamol, corticosteroids and oestroprogestins [34]. Medicinal plants are often used to alleviate jaundice, particularly in developing countries where access to qualified medical care is limited. Such treatments are generally not effective and may even exacerbate the course of the disease [66].

#### 1.1.2 Fulminant forms

Patients with a severe form should be treated in an intensive care unit. Treatment with N-acetyl-cysteine (a precursor of glutathione), especially if paracetamol has been taken, which is not uncommon during the prodromal phase, may be initiated in view of the favourable results of this treatment on transplant-free survival in severe acute hepatitis unrelated to paracetamol.

The most commonly used regimen consists of a loading dose of 150 mg/kg over 1 hour, followed by a maintenance infusion of 12.5 mg/kg/h over 4 hours and then 6.25 mg/kg/h until clinical and biological improvement is achieved. Spontaneous survival without transplantation increased from 30% to 52% [67].

The use of liver transplantation has transformed the prognosis of HAI, and must be discussed on a case-by-case basis. A large number of prognostic criteria, used alone or in combination, have been proposed in the literature.

Historically, the Clichy criteria and then the Kings College criteria are still used today to predict the need for transplantation [68]. The aim of resuscitation is to provide symptomatic management of the various associated organ failures in order to achieve spontaneous recovery of liver function or to bring the patient to transplantation under the best possible conditions.

In pregnant women, the effect of fetal extraction on the course of maternal infection has not been sufficiently studied [25].

Immunocompetent subjects spontaneously eliminate the virus without the need for antiviral treatment. However, a few authors have reported the use of ribavirin in acute fulminant forms of the disease or in subjects at risk of decompensating for underlying liver disease. In the absence of a control arm, it is not possible to establish the real benefit of this compound in these severe forms [69].

## 1.2 Antiviral treatment

No antiviral treatment has been evaluated in a controlled trial. INF alpha and ribavirin are the two antiviral treatments successfully prescribed for immunocompromised patients with chronic hepatitis E.

### 1.2.1 Chronic hepatitis

**- In solid organ transplant patients**

- Reducing immunosuppression by targeting T lymphocytes is the first line of treatment, eliminating the virus in a third of patients [44].

- Pegylated INF: This has been used successfully in liver transplant patients who remained viremic despite a reduction in immunosuppression, resulting in a sustained virological response (SVR) defined as undetectable viremia at least 6 months after stopping antiviral treatment. It cannot be used in heart, lung or kidney transplant patients because of bone marrow toxicity leading to tricytopenia and a risk of acute rejection [70].

- Ribavirin: effective as a single agent. In a French multicentre study, 59 solid organ transplant patients infected with HEV were treated with ribavirin. SVR was observed in 78% of patients. SVR was 74% in patients treated for 3 months or less and 85% in those treated for more than 3 months. The recommended dose is 12 mg/kg per day, or 600 to 800 mg per day for 3 to 6 months. The mechanism of action is still unknown. It has been suggested that the compound inhibits HEV replication by depletion of the guanosine triphosphate (GTP) pool [71].

There is no genotypic resistance to ribavirin, but a mutation that increases the replicative capacity of the virus has recently been identified. This mutation pre-exists treatment and is associated with higher viral loads, but has no impact on SVR. Given its oral administration, good tolerability and high efficacy, ribavirin, administered as a single agent, appears to be the drug of choice for the treatment of chronic hepatitis E. Virological monitoring after three months' treatment shows that the virus has been eradicated. Relapse may occur when treatment is stopped or when doses are reduced in response to the onset of severe anaemia [12].

- Sofosbuvir, a nucleotide analogue active on HCV RNA polymerase, has shown anti-HEV activity *in vitro* and could therefore be an alternative to ribavirin, given its favourable safety profile in transplant patients [72].

- New antiviral drugs active against HEV replication, such as the zinc salt and the nucleoside analogue 2-C-methylcytidine (2CMC) and calcineurin inhibitors, are promising therapies for the future [73].

- **In HIV-infected patients**

Antiretroviral treatment leading to a rise in $CD_4$ may allow HEV to be eliminated without specific treatment. Treatment regimens similar to those used in solid organ transplant patients have been used successfully [46].

- **In patients with haematological disease**

Pegylated INF alone for 3 months or ribavirin alone for 3 months have been used successfully to treat chronic HEV infections [45].

### 1.2.2 Acute hepatitis
In patients with underlying liver disease and a severe acute form (reduced prothrombin level, renal failure), the use of ribavirin led to rapid improvement in symptoms. In other immunocompetent patients without underlying liver disease but with severe acute infection with HEV 1 or 3, ribavirin has been used successfully. However, only isolated clinical cases have been reported and there have been no studies comparing the kinetics of viremia reduction and the outcome of patients with or without antiviral treatment [69].

### 1.2.3 Pregnant women
There is currently no established treatment for hepatitis E during pregnancy. In fact, the only treatments used to promote viral clearance, ribavirin with or without pegylated INF, are contraindicated during pregnancy. Modulation of the hormonal system is another treatment under investigation [25,69].

### 1.2.4 Extrahepatic manifestations
Cases of Guillain-Barré, myositis and membranoproliferative or extra-membranous glomerulopathies have been successfully treated with either interferon or ribavirin. Currently, despite the absence of large series, ribavirin treatment is proposed in cases of extrahepatic manifestations associated with HEV, whether these manifestations are observed in the acute or chronic phase of the infection [70].

## 2. Preventive treatment

The high endemicity of HEV in developing countries and the potential seriousness of the disease in pregnant women justify active prevention.

## 2.1 Collective measures

In developing countries, prevention is based mainly on the availability of drinking water and improved wastewater treatment, **with the** aim of reducing the number and scale of epidemics and isolated cases. In developed countries, water resources are generally of good quality [74].

### 2.1.1 Drinking water production

L he choice of drinking water treatment depends on the level of pollution of the resource. Simple chlorination is sufficient for groundwater, whereas a more complete treatment (advanced physical and chemical treatment and refining) is required for more polluted water. Free chlorine is the most common disinfectant, the easiest to use and the cheapest. It inactivates almost 100% of enterobacteria and viruses [74].

### 2.1.2 Wastewater treatment

Wastewater treatment is the first link in the fight against viral water pollution. Treatment takes place in three main stages. The primary stage involves mechanical removal of the coarse matter that sediments. In the secondary stage, organic matter is removed or destroyed biologically (viral abatement of 1 or 2 log units). The tertiary stage is used to protect areas of particular interest (bathing, shellfish farming, etc.) or catchment stations. Wastewater may therefore undergo various disinfection treatments (chlorination, $NH_2Cl$ or UV, or filtration processes), during which viral abatement is significant (4 log units) [74].

## 2.2 Individual measures

Individual prevention is based on strict compliance with non-specific hygiene rules to combat orofaecal peril.

## 2.3 Immunoprophylaxis

There is little information available on the administration of immunoglobulins, but the few existing studies suggest that immunoprophylaxis has not been successful in preventing infection, but only in alleviating the symptoms of hepatitis [10,76].

## 2.4 Vaccination

Vaccination is both an individual and collective prophylactic measure when used on a large scale, reducing the reservoir and quantity of viruses released into the environment. During major epidemics, health interventions and basic sanitation are not enough to rapidly stop the emergence of new infections. Much effort has gone into developing an HEV vaccine [21]. However, because of the difficulty of cultivating the virus, the production of a live attenuated vaccine or an inactivated vaccine was impossible, hence the use of recombinant HEV antigens [12].

At least 11 experimental vaccines have been evaluated in non-human primates. Two recombinant HEV vaccines have shown short-term efficacy[69].

- A vaccine against the recombinant HEV 1 protein (rHEV) had been tested on volunteers from the Nepalese army. All the volunteers who received the vaccine developed anti-HEV antibodies at a level greater than 20 Ul/ml one month after the third dose, but this immunity was retained in only 56.3% of them until the end of the study (804 days) [77].

Another vaccine called HEV 239 (Hecolin®) is a giant step forward in the prevention of hepatitis E in developing countries. It is a recombinant peptide from the ORF 2 region of an HEV 1 strain[78].

It is the only vaccine currently licensed and has been registered in China since 2011. However, it has not yet been approved in other countries [14]. The schedule adopted involves three doses: 0, 1 and 6 months in subjects aged between 16 and 65. The vaccine is more than 90% effective for 1 year after one dose and for 4.5 years after three doses. It is also well tolerated by pregnant women, and no major adverse effects or teratogenic effects on the foetus have been reported [79]. Although it is based on HEV 1, it has proved effective against HEV

4. Further studies are underway to determine whether it protects against HEV3, which is widespread in developed countries [10].

The cost-effectiveness of this vaccine has been debated. It costs approximately US$17.60 to US$41.70 per dose, less than the hepatitis A vaccine (price: US$23.21 per dose). Therefore, as vaccination can reduce the cost of hospitalisation and treatment, implementation of the HEV vaccine could be a cost-effective health intervention [80].

The WHO has not recommended its systematic inclusion in vaccination programmes for the general population, but suggests that it could be considered in endemic countries as part of a prevention programme to reduce the frequency of epidemics and possibly reduce the incidence of hepatitis E in high-risk groups: pregnant women and patients with chronic liver disease. In non-endemic regions, this vaccine is recommended for travellers planning to visit an endemic area [81].

The efficacy of the HEV 239 vaccine was tested in 12 pathogen-free rabbits, and the results of this study show that it is also effective and could possibly be extended to other animals, such as pigs [82].

The positive results obtained with HEV239 have encouraged researchers to develop vaccines that will provide combined protection against viruses sharing the same transmission route, such as Noroviruses. This bivalent vaccine is still under study [83].

# References


1. Hepatitis E.html. [Cited 30 Jan 2024]. Available from: https://www.who.int/news-room/fact- sheets/detail/hepatitis-e

2. Family: Hepeviridae |ICTV. [Cited 28 Apr 2024]. Available from : https://ictv.global/report/chapter/hepeviridae/hepeviridae

3. Luo et al - 2024 - Viral hepatitis E: Clinical manifestations, treatment. and prevention. Liver Research 8 (2024) 11e21.

4. Khuroo - 2023 - Discovery of Hepatitis E and Its Impact on Global. Khuroo, M.S. Discovery of Hepatitis E and Its Impact on Global Health: A Journey of 44 Years about an Incredible HumanInterest Story. Viruses 2023, 15, 1745. https://doi.org/10.3390/v15081745

5. Perez-Gracia MT. Current Knowledge on Hepatitis E. Journal of Clinical and Translational Hepatology. 15 June 2015;3(2):117−26.

6. Nicole Pavio, Xiang-Jin Meng, Virginie Doceul, Zoonotic origin of hepatitis E, Current Opinion in Virology, Volume 10, 2015, Pages 34-41, https://doi.org/10.1016/j.coviro.2014.12.006. pdf.

7. Hakim MS, Wang W, Bramer WM, Geng J, Huang F, de Man RA, et al. The global burden of hepatitis E outbreaks: a systematic review. Liver International. jan 2017;37(1):19−31.

8. Perez-Gracia MT. Acute, Chronic and Fulminant Hepatitis E: Ten Years of Experience (20042013). International Journal of Gastroenterology Disorders & Therapy [Internet]. 7 Jul 2014 [cited 11 Dec 2018];1(1). Available from: http://www.graphyonline.com/archives/IJGDT/2014/IJGDT- 102/

9. Pischke S, Hartl J, Pas SD, Lohse AW, Jacobs BC, Van der Eijk AA. Hepatitis E virus: Infection beyond the liver? Journal of Hepatology. May 2017;66(5):1082−95.

10. Pérez-Gracia MT, Suay-Garcia B, García M, Mateos-Lindemann ML. Hepatitis E: latest developments in knowledge. Future Microbiology. June 2016;11(6):789 − 808.

11. Aggarwal R. Diagnosis of hepatitis E. Nature Reviews Gastroenterology & Hepatology. jan 2013;10(1):24−33.

12. Melgaço JG, Gardinali NR, de Mello V da M, Leal M, Lewis-Ximenez LL, Pinto MA. Hepatitis E: Update on Prevention and Control. Biomed Res Int. 2018;2018:5769201.

13. Moucari R, Asselah T. Hepatitis E: will there soon be a vaccine? La Revue de Médecine Interne. August 2008;29(8):615–7.

14. WHO. Hepatitis E vaccine: WHO position paper, May 2015-- Recommendations. Vaccine. 12 Jan 2016;34(3):304–5.

15. Ditah et al - 2014 - Current epidemiology of hepatitis E virus infection in the United States: low seroprevalence in the National Health and Nutrition Evaluation Survey. Hepatology, 2014, vol. 60, no. 3, pp. 815-822. .pdf.

16. Ankcorn, M.J. and Tedder, R.S. (2017), Hepatitis E: the current state of play. Transfusion Med, 27: 84-95. https://doi-org.sndl1.arn.dz/10.1111/tme.12405

17. Aggarwal R, Naik SR. Hepatitis E: intrafamilial transmission versus waterborne spread. J Hepatol. Nov 1994;21(5):718–23.

18. Doceul V, Bagdassarian E, Demange A, Pavio N. Zoonotic Hepatitis E Virus: Classification, Animal Reservoirs and Transmission Routes. Viruses [Internet]. Oct 2016 [cited 16 Sep 2020];8(10). Available from: https://www.ncbi.nlm.nih.gov/pmc/articles/PMC5086606/

19. Khuroo M, Khuroo M, Khuroo N. Transmission of Hepatitis E Virus in Developing Countries. Viruses. 20 Sep 2016;8(9):253.

20. Chandra V, Taneja S, Kalia M, Jameel S. Molecular biology and pathogenesis of hepatitis E virus. Hepatitis E virus. 2008;14.

21. Purcell RH, Emerson SU. Hepatitis E: An emerging awareness of an old disease. Journal of Hepatology. 1 March 2008;48(3):494–503.

22. Dalton HR, Bendall R, Ijaz S, Banks M. Hepatitis E: an emerging infection in developed countries. The Lancet infectious diseases. 2008;8(11):698–709.

23. Srivastava R, Aggarwal R, Bhagat MR, Chowdhury A, Naik S. Alterations in natural killer cells and natural killer T cells during acute viral hepatitis E: NK and NKT cells in hepatitis E. Journal of Viral Hepatitis. Dec 2008;15(12):910 – 6.

24. Prabhu SB, Gupta P, Durgapal H, Rath S, Gupta SD, Acharya SK, et al. Study of cellular immune response against hepatitis E virus (HEV). Journal of viral hepatitis. 2011;18(8):587 – 94.

25. Pérez-Gracia MT, Suay-Garcia B, Mateos-Lindemann ML. Hepatitis E and pregnancy: current state. Reviews in Medical Virology. may 2017;27(3):e1929.

26. Bose PD, Das BC, Kumar A, Gondal R, Kumar D, Kar P. High viral load and deregulation of the progesterone receptor signaling pathway: association with hepatitis E-related poor pregnancy outcome. Journal of hepatology. 2011;54(6):1107–13.

27. M B. Prevalence and severity of acute viral hepatitis and fulminant hepatitis during pregnancy: A prospective study from north india. Indian Journal of Medical Microbiology. 7 Jan 2003;21(3):184.

28. Kamar N, Garrouste C, Haagsma EB, Garrigue V, Pischke S, Chauvet C, et al. Factors Associated With Chronic Hepatitis in Patients With Hepatitis E Virus Infection Who Have Received Solid Organ Transplants. Gastroenterology. May 1, 2011;140(5):1481 –9.

29. Lee GH, Tan BH, Chi-Yuan Teo E, Lim SG, Dan YY, Wee A, et al. Chronic Infection With Camelid Hepatitis E Virus in a Liver Transplant Recipient Who Regularly Consumes Camel Meat and Milk. Gastroenterology. feb 2016;150(2):355-357.e3.

30. Krawczynski K. Hepatitis E. Hepatology. 1993;17(5):932–41.

31. Peron JM, Danjoux M, Kamar N, Missoury R, Poirson H, Vinel JP, et al. Liver histology in patients with sporadic acute hepatitis E: a study of 11 patients from South-West France. Virchows Archiv. 2007;450(4):405–10.

32. Aggarwal R. Clinical presentation of hepatitis E. Virus Research. Oct 2011;161(1):15–22.

33. Kamar N, Bendall RP, Peron JM, Cintas P, Prudhomme L, Mansuy JM, et al. Hepatitis E Virus and Neurologic Disorders. Emerg Infect Dis. Feb 2011;17(2):173–9.

34. Goel A, Aggarwal R. Advances in hepatitis E - II: Epidemiology, clinical manifestations, treatment and prevention. Expert Review of Gastroenterology & Hepatology. sept 2016;10(9):1065–74.

35. Couturier É. Hepatitis E: summary of human epidemiology. Bulletin épidémiologique Spécial zoonoses. 2010;38:20−1.

36. Lhomme S. Hepatitis E virus. Biologie médicale. :11.

37. Irshad M. Hepatitis E Virus: An Update on Its Molecular, Clinical and Epidemiological Characteristics. INT. 1999;42(4):252−62.

38. Jilani N, Das BC, Husain SA, Baweja UK, Chattopadhya D, Gupta RK, et al. Hepatitis E virus infection and fulminant hepatic failure during pregnancy. Journal of gastroenterology and hepatology. 2007;22(5):676−82.

39. PÉron JM, Mansuy JM, Poirson H, Bureau C, Dupuis E, Alric L, et al. Hepatitis E is an autochthonous disease in industrialized countries. Gastroentérologie Clinique et Biologique. May 2006;30(5):757−62.

40. Kumar M, Sharma BC, Sarin SK. Hepatitis E virus as an etiology of acute exacerbation of previously unrecognized asymptomatic patients with hepatitis B virus-related chronic liver disease. Journal of gastroenterology and hepatology. 2008;23(6):883−7.

41. Kumar Acharya S, Kumar Sharma P, Singh R, Kumar Mohanty S, Madan K, Kumar Jha J, et al. Hepatitis E virus (HEV) infection in patients with cirrhosis is associated with rapid decompensation and death. Journal of Hepatology. March 2007;46(3):387−94.

42. Patra S, Kumar A, Trivedi SS, Puri M, Sarin SK. Maternal and fetal outcomes in pregnant women with acute hepatitis E virus infection. Annals of internal medicine. 2007;147(1):28−33.

43. Stoszek SK, Abdel-Hamid M, Saleh DA, Kafrawy SE, Narooz S, Hawash Y, et al. High prevalence of hepatitis E antibodies in pregnant Egyptian women. Trans R Soc Trop Med Hyg. 1 Feb 2006;100(2):95−101.

44. Kamar N, Selves J, Mansuy JM, Ouezzani L, Péron JM, Guitard J, et al. Hepatitis E Virus and Chronic Hepatitis in Organ-Transplant Recipients. New England Journal of Medicine. 21 Feb 2008;358(8):811 −7.

45. Tavitian S, Péron JM, Huynh A, Mansuy JM, Ysebaert L, Huguet F, et al. Hepatitis E virus excretion can be prolonged in patients with hematological malignancies. Journal of Clinical Virology. 2010;49(2):141−4.

46. Dalton HR, Bendall RP, Keane FE, Tedder RS, Ijaz S. Persistent carriage of hepatitis E virus in patients with HIV infection. New England Journal of Medicine. 2009;361(10):1025-7.

47. Grewal P, Kamili S, Motamed D. Chronic hepatitis E in an immunocompetent patient: a case report. Hepatology. 2014;59(1):347 – 8.

48. Tallon G. Chronic hepatitis E in an immunocompetent patient. Gastoenteology and Hepatology. 2011;34(8):398-400.

49. van den Berg B, van der Eijk AA, Pas SD, Hunter JG, Madden RG, Tio-Gillen AP, et al. Guillain-Barré syndrome associated with preceding hepatitis E virus infection. Neurology. Feb 11, 2014;82(6):491 -7.

50. Bhagat S, Wadhawan M, Sud R, Arora A. Hepatitis viruses causing pancreatitis and hepatitis: a case series and review of literature. Pancreas. May 2008;36(4):424-7.

51. Colson P, Payraudeau E, Leonnet C, De Montigny S, Villeneuve L, Motte A, et al. Severe thrombocytopenia associated with acute hepatitis E virus infection. J Clin Microbiol. Jul 2008;46(7):2450-2.

52. Serratrice J, Disdier P, Colson P, Ene N, de Roux CS, Weiller PJ. Acute polyarthritis revealing hepatitis E. Clin Rheumatol. Nov 2007;26(11):1973-5.

53. Myara A, Imbert-Bismut F, Piton A, Schilliger O, Antoniotti G. [Role of biology in the follow up of viral hepatitis]. Ann Biol Clin (Paris). Oct 1998;56(5):527 – 37.

54. Krawczynski K, Meng XJ, Rybczynska J. Pathogenetic elements of hepatitis E and animal models of HEV infection. Virus Research. 1 Oct 2011;161(1):78-83.

55. Walsh SR. 180 - Hepatitis E Virus. Hepatitis E Virus. :15.

56. Abravanel F, Chapuy-Regaud S, Lhomme S, Miedougé M, Peron JM, Alric L, et al. Performance of anti-HEV assays for diagnosing acute hepatitis E in immunocompromised patients. Journal of Clinical Virology. dec 2013;58(4):624 – 8.

57. Mansuy JM, Peron JM, Bureau C, Alric L, Vinel JP, Izopet J. Immunologically silent autochthonous acute hepatitis E virus infection in

France. J Clin Microbiol. Feb 2004;42(2):912-3.

58. Teshale EH. Hepatitis E: Epidemiology and prevention. World Journal of Hepatology. 2011;3(12):285.

59. Hyams C, Mabayoje DA, Copping R, Maranao D, Patel M, Labbett W, et al. Serological cross reactivity to CMV and EBV causes problems in the diagnosis of acute hepatitis E virus infection. J Med Virol. March 2014;86(3):478 – 83.

60. Shrestha AC, Flower RLP, Seed CR, Stramer SL, Faddy HM. A Comparative Study of Assay Performance of Commercial Hepatitis E Virus Enzyme-Linked Immunosorbent Assay Kits in Australian Blood Donor Samples. Journal of Blood Transfusion. 2016;2016:1-6.

61. Nicand E, Grandadam M, Teyssou R, Rey JL, Buisson Y. Viraemia and faecal shedding of HEV in symptom-free carriers. Lancet. 6 Jan 2001;357(9249):68-9.

62. Kamar N, Bendall R, Legrand-Abravanel F, Xia NS, Ijaz S, Izopet J, et al. Hepatitis E. Lancet. 30 June 2012;379(9835):2477-88.

63. Zhang JZ, Im SWK, Lau SH, Chau TN, Lai ST, Ng SP, et al. Occurrence of hepatitis E virus IgM, low avidity IgG serum antibodies, and viremia in sporadic cases of non-A, -B, and -C acute hepatitis. J Med Virol. Jan 2002;66(1):40 – 8.

64. Debing Y, Moradpour D, Neyts J, Gouttenoire J. Update on hepatitis E virology: Implications for clinical practice. Journal of Hepatology. Jul 2016;65(1):200-12.

65. Renou C, Nicand E, Pariente A, Cadranel JF, Pavio N. When to look for and how to diagnose indigenous hepatitis E? Clinical and Biological Gastroenterology. 1 Oct 2009;33(10, Supplement):F27-35.

40. Bernuau JR, Durand F. Herbal medicines in acute viral hepatitis: a ticket for more trouble. Eur J Gastroenterol Hepatol. March 2008;20(3):161 -3.

41. Lee WM, Hynan LS, Rossaro L, Fontana RJ, Stravitz RT, Larson AM, et al. Intravenous N- acetylcysteine improves transplant-free survival in early stage non-acetaminophen acute liver failure. Gastroenterology.

2009;137(3):856-64.

42. Bernal W, Auzinger G, Dhawan A, Wendon J. Acute liver failure. The Lancet. 2010;376(9736):190-201.

43. Donnelly MC, Scobie L, Crossan CL, Dalton H, Hayes PC, Simpson KJ. Review article: hepatitis E-a concise review of virology, epidemiology, clinical presentation and therapy. Alimentary Pharmacology & Therapeutics. july 2017;46(2):126–41.

44. Kamar N, Rostaing L, Abravanel F, Garrouste C, Esposito L, Cardeau-Desangles I, et al. Pegylated interferon-a for treating chronic hepatitis E virus infection after liver transplantation. Clinical Infectious Diseases. 2010;50(5):e30 – 3.

45. Kamar N, Izopet J, Tripon S, Bismuth M, Hillaire S, Dumortier J, et al. Ribavirin for chronic hepatitis E virus infection in transplant recipients. N Engl J Med. March 20, 2014;370(12):1111 –20.

46. Thi VLD, Debing Y, Wu X, Rice CM, Neyts J, Moradpour D, et al. Sofosbuvir inhibits hepatitis E virus replication in vitro and results in an additive effect when combined with ribavirin. Gastroenterology. 2016;150(1):82-5.

47. Garbuglia AR, Scognamiglio P, Petrosillo N, Mastroianni CM, Sordillo P, Gentile D, et al. Hepatitis E Virus Genotype 4 Outbreak, Italy, 2011. Emerg Infect Dis. Jan 2013;19(1):110–4.

48. WHO | Waterborne hepatitis E epidemics: identification, investigation and control [Internet]. WHO. [cited 22 Dec 2018]. Available from: http://www.who.int/hepatitis/publications/HepE- manual/en/

49. Nelson KE, Heaney CD, Labrique AB, Kmush BL, Krain LJ. Hepatitis E: prevention and treatment. Current Opinion in Infectious Diseases. oct 2016;29(5):478 – 85.

50. Arankalle VA, Chadha MS, Dama BM, Tsarev SA, Purcell RH, Banerjee K. Role of immune serum globulins in pregnant women during an

epidemic of hepatitis E. J Viral Hepat. May 1998;5(3):199–204.

77. Shrestha MP, Scott RM, Joshi DM, Mammen MP, Thapa GB, Thapa N, et al. Safety and efficacy of a recombinant hepatitis E vaccine. N Engl J Med. March 1, 2007;356(9):895 –903.

78. Ankcorn MJ, Tedder RS. Hepatitis E: the current state of play: Hepatitis E. Transfusion Medicine. Apr 2017;27(2):84–95.

79. Wu T, Zhu FC, Huang SJ, Zhang XF, Wang ZZ, Zhang J, et al. Safety of the hepatitis E vaccine for pregnant women: a preliminary analysis. Hepatology. 2012;55(6):2038 – 2038.

80. Zhu FC, Zhang J, Zhang XF, Zhou C, Wang ZZ, Huang SJ, et al. Efficacy and safety of a recombinant hepatitis E vaccine in healthy adults: a large-scale, randomised, double-blind placebo- controlled, phase 3 trial. The Lancet. 2010;376(9744):895-902.

81. Harmanci H, Duclos P, Rodriguez Hernandez CA, Meek A, Balakrishnan MR, Kumar Arora N, et al. World Health Organization approaches to evaluating the potential use and quality of Hepatitis E vaccine. In: Open forum infectious diseases. Oxford University Press; 2014.

82. Liu P, jie Du R, Wang L, Han J, Liu L, lin Zhang Y, et al. Management of hepatitis E virus (HEV) zoonotic transmission: protection of rabbits against HEV challenge following immunization with HEV 239 vaccine. PLoS One. 2014;9(1):e87600.

83. Wang L, Cao D, Wei C, Meng XJ, Jiang X, Tan M. A dual vaccine candidate against norovirus and hepatitis E virus. Vaccine. 16 Jan 2014;32(4):445 – 52.

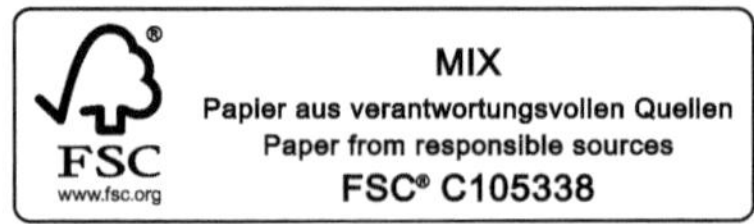

Printed by Books on Demand GmbH, Norderstedt / Germany